Published By Adam Gilbin

@ Steven Swim

Sirt Food Diet: Plan Your Weight Loss With Easy

and Delicious Recipes Rich in Sirt Foods

All Right RESERVED

ISBN 978-1-990666-68-1

TABLE OF CONTENTS

Turmeric Roasted Potatoes & Cauliflower

Ingredients:

- 10 baby potatoes, peeled and washed

- ⅓ cup (80ml) hot mustard

- 1 tbsp turmeric

- ⅓ cup (80ml) olive oil

- 1 medium cauliflower head, cut into florets

- Salt

- Pepper

Directions:

1. Combine the turmeric with the mustard and olive oil in a bowl.

2. Preheat your oven to 390F/195C.

3. Place the cauliflower and potatoes (interchangeably) in a baking tray lined with

parchment paper and brush with the mustard and turmeric mixture. Season with extra salt and pepper.

4. Bake in the oven for approx. 40 minutes.

Pasta With Creamy Kale Sauce

Ingredients:

- 1 tbsp pesto sauce

- ½ cup (120ml) soy or vegetable cream

- 1 tbsp parmesan, shredded

- 2 tbsp olive oil

- 1 ½ cup (140g) whole-wheat penne pasta

- 4 cups (1 liter) water

- 1 bunch kale, roughly chopped

- 1 small red onion, chopped

- Salt

- Pepper

Directions:

1. Cook the penne pasta for 12-15 minutes in salted boiling water or according to package Directions:.
2. Remove from the heat, drain, and set aside.
3. Meanwhile, heat the olive oil in a pan and saute the onion for 2 minutes.
4. Add the chopped kale and saute until wilted for 2-3 minutes.
5. Add the pesto and soy cream to the pan and cook for 2-3 minutes.
6. Finally add the cooked penne pasta, salt, and pepper to taste, the parmesan, and stir.
7. Serve warm.

Meatloaf Pita Sandwich

Ingredients:

- 5og rocket

- 1 stalk parsley/lovage

- 1 tablespoon of extra virgin olive oil

- ½ cup of shredded, mozzarella cheese/ feta cheese

- 1 red onion, chopped

- 1 tomato, diced

- 1 meatloaf

- 1 whole pita meat, pita bread

- Salt

- Pepper

- 1 tablespoon of lemon juice

Directions:

1. Microwave the meatloaf and cut it into pieces. Divide into two
2. Mix the pepper, onion, tomatoes, salt, parsley/lovage, rocket, lemon juice, olive oil. Add the cheese and stir.
3. Cut the pita bread into 2. Fill each half with the meatloaf and salad dressing. Serve.

Haitian Kale Shrimp Stew

Ingredients:

- 3 cups kale leaves

- 1 tsp. dried red pepper flakes (to taste).

- 4 whole cloves (discard after cooking)

- 2 cups fish broth

- 1 cup tomato paste.

- 1 lime – juice only & 1/8 ground cloves

- 2 cups chopped onions

- 2 tbsp. olive oil

- Salt, black pepper to taste

- 4 pounds shrimp

Directions:

1. Put Ingredients: in the slow cooker. Cover, & cook on low for 8 hours.

Kale Chicken Jambalaya

Ingredients:

- 1 tsp. dried red pepper flakes (to taste).

- 3 cups kale & 1 cup mushrooms

- 1 cup tomato paste & 1 cup chicken broth

- 1 cup corn & 1 cup chopped carrot

- 1 cup chopped onions & 2 minced garlic cloves

- 2 tbsp. olive oil & 1 tsp. turmeric

- Salt, black pepper to taste

- 3 pounds cubed chicken & 1 pound shrimp

Directions:

1. Put Ingredients: in the slow cooker. Cover, & cook on low for 8 hours.

Mexican Bell Pepper Filled With Egg:

Ingredients:

- ¼ teaspoon Paprika powder

- ½ pieces Avocado

- 1 piece green peppers

- 2 tablespoon fresh coriander

- 1 tablespoon Coconut oil

- 4 pieces Egg

- 1 piece Tomato

- 1 pinch Chili flakes

- ¼ teaspoon Ground cumin

Directions:

1. Cut the tomatoes and avocado into cubes and finely chop the fresh coriander.

2. Melt the coconut oil in a pan over medium heat, beat the eggs in the pan, and add the tomato cubes.
3. Keep stirring until the eggs solidify and season with chili, caraway, paprika, pepper, and salt.
4. Finally, add the avocado.
5. Place the egg mixture in the pepper halves and garnish with fresh coriander.

Frittata With Spring Onions And Asparagus:

Ingredients:

- 100 g Asparagus tips

- 4 pieces Spring onions

- 1 teaspoon Tarragon

- 1 pinch Chilli flakes

- 5 pieces Egg

- 80 ml (3 fl. Oz.) Almond milk

- 2 tablespoon Coconut oil

- 1 clove Garlic

Directions:

1. Preheat the oven to 220°C (430°F).
2. Squeeze the garlic and finely chop the spring onions.

3. Whisk the eggs with the almond milk and season with salt and pepper.
4. Melt 1 tablespoon of coconut oil in a medium-sized cast iron pan and briefly fry the onion and garlic with the asparagus.
5. Remove the vegetables from the pan and melt the remaining coconut oil in the pan.
6. Pour in the egg mixture and half of the entire vegetable.
7. Place the pan in the oven for 15 minutes until the egg has solidified.
8. Then take the pan out of the oven and pour the rest of the egg with the vegetables into the pan.
9. Place the pan in the oven again for 15 minutes until the egg is nice and loose.
10. Sprinkle the tarragon and chili flakes on the dish before serving.

Fragrant Asian Hotpot

Ingredients:

- 500ml chicken stock, fresh or made with 1 cube

- ½ peeled carrot, and cut into sticks

- 50g beansprouts

- 100g raw tiger prawns

- 100g firm tofu, chopped

- 50g broccoli, cut into tiny florets

- 50g rice noodles, boiled according to packet 1 tsp. tomato purée

- 10g Small handful parsley, finely chopped stalks

- 10g Small handful coriander, finely chopped stalks

- Juice of ½ lemon

- 1 crushed star anise (or ¼ tsp. ground anise)

- 20g sushi ginger, finely chopped

- 50g boiled water chestnuts, drained

- 1 tbsp. better-quality miso paste

Directions:

1. Place the tomato purée, star anise, parsley stalks, coriander stalks, lime juice and chicken stock in a large pan and bring to a simmer for almost 10 minutes.

2. Add the carrot, broccoli, prawns, tofu, noodles and water chestnuts and simmer gently until the prawns are cooked through. Remove from the heat and stir in the sushi ginger and miso paste.

3. Serve sprinkled with the parsley and coriander leaves.

Butternut Squash, Date And Tagline Lamb

Ingredients:

- 2 teaspoons of cumin seeds

- 2 teaspoons turmeric, grounded

- ½ teaspoon salt

- 800g lamb neck fillet, sliced to 2cm chunks

- 100g Medjool dates, chopped and pitted

- 500g butternut squash, finely chopped to 1cm cubes

- 2 tbsp. of coriander (and extra for garnishing)

- 400g chopped tomatoes and a half cup of water

- 400g tin chickpeas, boiled and drained

- 2 tbsp. virgin olive oil

- 2cm ginger, chopped

- 1 red onion, cut

- 3 cloves of garlic, crushed or grated

- 1 teaspoon red chilli flakes (according to your taste)

- 1 cinnamon stick

- Couscous, Buckwheat, rice or flatbreads for serving

Directions:

1. Oven preheated to 140C. In a large oven-proof pan or a cast iron casserole plate, add around 2 teaspoons of olive oil.

2. Attach the cut onion and cook onto a low flame until the onions are cooked but not dark, with the lid on for around 5 minutes.
3. Attach the dried ginger and garlic, cumin, cinnamon, chilli and turmeric.
4. Mix well, and cook the lid off for one more minute. If it becomes too dry add a drop of water.
5. After that, add in chunks of the lamb.
6. Mix well to cover the meat in spices and onions, and then apply butter, chopped tomatoes and dates, plus around half a cup of water (100-200ml).
7. Take tagine to boil, and then place the cover on and position for about 1 hour and 15 minutes in your preheated oven.
8. Take out from the oven when the tagine is prepared, and mix it through chopped coriander.

9. Present with couscous, basmati rice or
    flatbreads.

Buckwheat Pancakes With Strawberries, Dark Chocolate Sauce

Ingredients:

For the pancakes you will need:

- 1 large egg

- 1 tbsp extra virgin olive oil, for cooking

- 350ml milk

- 150g buckwheat flour

For the chocolate sauce

- 100g dark chocolate (85 percent cocoa solids)

- 85ml milk

- 1 tbsp double cream

- 1 tbsp extra virgin olive oil

Directions:

1. To make the pancake batter, place all of the Ingredients: apart from the olive oil in a mixer and mix till you have a smooth batter. It ought to not be too thick or too runny. (You can save any excess batter in an airtight container for up to 5 days in your fridge. Be sure to mix well prior to using once again.).

2. To make the chocolate sauce, melt the chocolate in a heatproof bowl over a pan of simmering water. When melted, mix in the milk, whisking thoroughly and after that include the double cream and olive oil. You can keep the sauce warm by leaving the water in the pan simmering on a very low heat till your pancakes are ready.

3. To make the pancakes heat a heavy-bottomed fry pan up until it begins to smoke, then include the olive oil.

4. Put some of the batter into the centre of the pan, then tip the excess batter around it up

until you have covered the whole surface, you may have to include a bit more batter to achieve this. You will only require to prepare the pancake for 1 minute or so on each side if your pan is hot enough.

5. As soon as you can see it going brown around the edges utilize a spatula to loosen up the pancake around its edge, then flip it over. Attempt to flip in one action to avoid breaking it.

6. Cook for a further minute approximately on the other side and transfer to a plate.

7. Place some strawberries in the centre and roll up the pancake. Continue till you have made as numerous pancakes as required.

8. Spoon over a generous amount of sauce and spray over some sliced walnuts.

9. You might find that your very first efforts are too fat or break down but once you discover the consistency of your batter that works

finest for you and you get your strategy improved you'll be making them like an expert. Practice makes best in this case.

Blueberry Banana Pancakes With Chunky Apple Compote And Golden Tumeric Latte

Ingredients:

For the Blueberry Banana Pancakes

- 2 tsp baking powder

- ¼ teaspoon salt

- 25g blueberries

- 6 bananas

- 6 eggs

- 150g rolled oats

For the Chunky Apple Compote

- 5 dates (pitted)

- 1 tablespoon lemon juice

- 1/4 teaspoon cinnamon powder

- 2 apples

- Pinch salt

For the Golden Turmeric Latte

- 3 cups coconut milk

- 1 teaspoon turmeric powder

- 1 teaspoon cinnamon powder

- 1 teaspoon raw honey

- Pinch of black pepper (increases absorption)

- Tiny piece of fresh, peeled ginger root

- Pinch of cayenne pepper (optional)

Directions:

For the Blueberry Banana Pancakes

1. Pop the rolled oats in a high-speed mixer and pulse for 1 minute or until an oat flour has formed.

2. Suggestion: make sure your mixer is very dry prior to doing this or else everything will become soaked!

3. Now add the bananas, eggs, baking powder and salt to the blender and pulse for 2 minutes up until a smooth batter forms.

4. Transfer the mixture to a large bowl and fold in the blueberries. Delegate rest for 10 minutes whilst the baking powder activates.

5. To make your pancakes, add a dollop of butter (this helps to make them really delicious and crispy!) to your fry pan on a medium-high heat.

6. Include a couple of spoons of the blueberry pancake mix and fry for until perfectly golden

on the bottom side. Toss the pancake to fry the opposite.

For the Chunky Apple Compote

1. Core and rough chop your apples.
2. Pop whatever in a food mill, together with 2 tablespoons of water and a pinch of salt.
3. Pulse to form your chunky apple compote.

For the Golden Turmeric Latte

1. Blend all Ingredients: in a high-speed blender till smooth.
2. Pour into a small pan and heat for 4 minutes over medium heat until hot however not boiling.

Avocado With Pine Nuts

Ingredients:

- Salt and pepper

- 1 tbsp pine nuts

- 1 lime

- Olive oil

- 1 pear

- 1 avocado

Directions:

1. Wash the ripe avocado with the pear, deseed, cut into long pieces and place alternately on a large plate.
2. Sprinkle lime juice over the fruit.
3. Roast the pine nuts in a pan for 2 minutes.
4. Add the kernels as well.

5. Season with salt and pepper. Serve.

Pears With Pine Nuts And Goat Cheese

Ingredients:

- 100 g of goat cheese

- Salt and pepper

- 1 tbsp chives

- 2 tbsp pine nuts

- 2 pears

- 1 ½ tbsp honey (liquid)

- 2 tsp lemon juice

Directions:

1. Wash, core and halve the pears.

2. Remove the core from the center of the pear using a ball-type cookie cutter. (also works with a spoon)

3. Roast the kernels in a pan. Then leave to cool in a bowl.

4. Mix the honey with the lemon juice and the cheese and season with salt and pepper.

5. Place the pears on a large plate and fill with the goat cheese. Scatter over the chives with the pine nuts.

6. If necessary, drizzle some honey over the pears.

Raspberry Greens Smoothie

Ingredients:

- 2 tbsp. lime juice

- 1 cup coconut milk

- 1 handful leafy greens

- 1 cup raspberries (frozen)

Directions:

1. Add all Ingredients: to a high-power blender and pulse until smooth.
2. Pour the smoothie into two glasses and serve immediately.
3. It can be stored in the refrigerator in an airtight container for up to 3 days.

Scalloped Eggplant

Ingredients:

- 1/2 cup soymilk

- 2 cups buckwheat breadcrumbs

- 1/2 tsp. Paprika

- 1 tsp. Turmeric

- 1/4 tsp. Cayenne

- Eggplant, diced

- 2 cups mushrooms, thinly chopped

- 1 red onion, thinly chopped

- 1 bell pepper, thinly chopped

- 3 tbsp. Olive oil

Directions:

1. Preheat oven to 350°F. In a skillet, sauté the eggplant, mushrooms, onion, and bell pepper in the oil until the eggplant becomes golden, about 10 minutes

2. Mix the milk, paprika, turmeric, cayenne, salt, and pepper with breadcrumbs.

3. Put the veggie mix on a tray, cover with the breadcrumb mixture and bake for 25 minutes.

Salmon With Turmeric And Chili

Ingredients:

- 1 garlic clove, finely chopped

- 1 bird's eye chili, finely chopped

- 150 g celery cut into 2cm lengths

- 1 teaspoon mild curry powder

- 130 g tomato, cut into 8 wedges

- 100 ml chicken or vegetable stock

- 1 tablespoon chopped parsley

- Skinned salmon

- 1 teaspoon extra virgin olive oil

- 1 teaspoon ground turmeric

- ¼ lemon, juiced

- 40 g red onion, finely chopped

- 60 g tinned green lentils

Directions:

1. Heat the oven to 200°C/gas mark 6.
2. Start with the spicy celery. Heat a frying pan over medium-low heat; add the olive oil, then the onion, garlic, ginger, chili, and celery.
3. Fry gently for 2-3 minutes or until softened but not colored, then add the curry powder and cook for another minute.
4. Add the tomatoes, then the stock and lentils, and simmer gently for 10 minutes.
5. You may want to increase or decrease the cooking time depending on how crunchy you like your celery.
6. Meanwhile, mix the turmeric, oil, and lemon juice and rub over the salmon.
7. Place on a baking tray and bake for 8-10 minutes.

8. To finish, stir the parsley through the celery and serve with the salmon.

Pesto-Parmesan Sauce

Ingredients:

- 1/2 teaspoon salt

- 1 teaspoon pepper

- 1 garlic clove, minced

- 1 ounce grated Parmesan cheese

- Serve over cooked vegetables.

- 2 cups firmly packed fresh basil leaves, chopped

- 1 tablespoon plus 1 teaspoon olive oil

Directions:

1. In a blender container, combine all Ingredients: except cheese and process until smooth, stopping the motor when necessary

to scrape the mixture down from sides of the container.

2. Transfer sauce to a small bowl and stir In cheese; serve immediately or cover and refrigerate.

3. When ready to use, bring to room temperature.

Red Clam Sauce

Ingredients:

- 2 teaspoons basil leaves

- 1/2 teaspoon salt

- Dash each oregano leaves and pepper

- 8 ounces drained canned minced clams

- 2 tablespoons chopped fresh parsley

- Serve over cooked linguini or spaghetti.

- 2 teaspoons olive oil 1/2 cup chopped onion

- 2 garlic cloves, minced

- 3 cups canned Italian tomatoes, crushed

- 1 cup bottled clam juice

Directions:

1. In 1/2-quart saucepan heat oil; add onion and garlic and saute for about 2 minutes.
2. Add remaining Ingredients: except for clams and parsley and bring to a boil.
3. Reduce heat and let simmer, occasionally stirring, for about 15 minutes.
4. Add clams and parsley and cook until thoroughly heated, about 3 minutes longer.

Split-Pea Soup

Ingredients:

- 2 cloves of garlic, minced

- 1 bay leaf

- ½ tsp nutmeg

- ½ tsp cayenne pepper

- 2 tbsp olive oil

- 4 cups (1 liter) vegetable broth

- 1 ½ cups (300g) split-peas, soaked in water

- 1 large carrot, sliced

- 1 medium red onion, sliced

- Salt

- Pepper

Directions:

1. Heat the olive oil in a pot and add the onion, garlic, and carrots. Saute for 2-3 minutes.
2. Add the vegetable broth and bring to a boil.
3. Add the split peas, bay leaf, and spices and cook cover over medium to low heat for 40 minutes.
4. Serve warm.

Roasted Green Beans & Pork Sausage

Ingredients:

- 3 spicy sausage links, thickly cut

- A drizzle of olive oil

- 1 tbsp sesame seeds

- 1 pound (500g) frozen or fresh green beans, trimmed

- Salt

- Pepper

- Greasing spray

Directions:

1. Preheat your oven to 400F/200C.
2. Place the green beans and sausage slices on a greased baking tray, drizzle with olive oil and

add the sesame seeds on top of the green beans.

3. Bake in the oven for 20 minutes.

Coronation Chicken Salad

Ingredients:

- 200g Cooked chicken breast

- 12 Walnut halves, finely chopped

- 2 Medjool date, finely chopped

- 40g red onion, diced

- 2 Bird's eye chilli

- 80g Rocket

- 150g of natural yoghurt

- 1/2 lemon

- 2 teaspoons of Coriander, chopped

- 2 teaspoons of Ground turmeric

- 1 teaspoon of Mild curry powder

Directions:

1. In a cup, mix the lemon juice, yoghurt, coriander and spices.
2. Add the remainder of the Ingredients: and serve on a rocket bed.

Baked Potatoes With Spicy Chickpea Stew

Ingredients:

- 2 tablespoons cumin seeds

- 2 tablespoons turmeric

- water

- 2 x 400g tins chopped tomatoes

- 2 tablespoons unsweetened cocoa powder

- 2 x 400g tins chickpeas/kidney beans

- 2 fresh peppers, chopped

- 2 tablespoons parsley

- 4 baking potatoes, pricked

- 2 tablespoons of olive oil

- 2 red onions, finely chopped

- 4 cloves garlic, grated

- 2cm ginger, grated

- 1 teaspoon of chilli flakes

- Salt and pepper to taste (optional)

- Side salad (optional)

Directions:

1. Preheat the oven to 200C and get all your Ingredients: ready. Put your potatoes in the oven and cook until they are done at least for 1 hour.

2. Cook the olive oil and chopped red onion using a large wide saucepan for 5 minutes while covering it until the onions are soft but not brown.

3. Add the ginger, cumin, garlic, and chilli and cook for extra 1 minute on a low heat before adding the turmeric. Add a very small splash

of water to prevent the pan from getting very dry and cook for another minute.

4. Add in the tomatoes, cocoa powder, yellow pepper, and chickpeas with the chickpea water and simmer on a low heat for 45 minutes to enable the sauce to become thick and unctuous.

5. Stir in the parsley, salt and pepper to taste and serve the stew on top of the baked potatoes, and with a simple side salad if you wish.

Kale, Quinoa And Beans Stew

Ingredients:

- 2 cups tomatoes, chopped

- Salt, black pepper and ground cumin to taste

- 2 cups chicken or vegetable stock

- 1 cup quinoa

- 2 cups raw kidney beans

- 2 cups chopped onions

- 2 cups chopped kale

- 1 cup sliced carrot

- 2 tbsp. olive oil

Directions:

1. Put Ingredients: in the slow cooker. Cover, & cook on low for 7 to 9 hours.

50

Vegetarian Paleo Ratatouille

Ingredients:

- 2 tablespoon Olive oil

- 1 piece Eggplant

- 1 piece Zucchini

- 1 piece hot peppers

- 1 teaspoon dried thyme

- 200 g (7 oz.) Tomato cubes (can)

- ½ pieces Onion

- 2 cloves Garlic

- ¼ teaspoon dried oregano

- ¼ TL Chili flakes

Directions:

1. Preheat the oven to 180°C (350°F) and lightly grease a round or oval shape.

2. Finely chop the onion and garlic.

3. Mix the tomato cubes with garlic, onion, oregano and chili flakes, season with salt and pepper, and put on the bottom of the baking dish.

4. Use a mandolin, a cheese slicer or a sharp knife to cut the eggplant, zucchini and hot pepper into very thin slices.

5. Put the vegetables in a bowl (make circles, start at the edge and work inside).

6. Drizzle the remaining olive oil on the vegetables and sprinkle with thyme, salt, and pepper.

7. Cover the baking dish with a piece of parchment paper and bake in the oven for 45 to 55 minutes.

8. Enjoy it!

Lentil & Greens Soup Corn And Black Bean Soup

Ingredients:

- 1 teaspoon ground turmeric

- ¼ teaspoon red pepper flakes

- 1 (14½-ounce) can diced tomatoes

- 1 cup red lentils, rinsed

- 5½ cups water

- 2 cups fresh mustard greens, chopped

- Salt and ground black pepper, to taste

- 2 tablespoons fresh lemon juice

- 1 tablespoon olive oil

- 2 carrots, peeled and chopped

- 2 celery stalks, chopped

- 1 medium yellow onion, chopped

- 3 garlic cloves, minced

- 1½ teaspoon ground cumin

Directions:

1. Heat olive oil in a large pan over medium heat and sauté the carrots, celery, and onion for about 5–6 minutes.

2. Add the garlic and spices and sauté for about 1 minute.

3. Add the tomatoes and cook for about 2–3 minutes.

4. Stir in the lentils and water and bring to a boil.

5. Now, reduce the heat to low and simmer, covered for about 35 minutes.

6. Stir in greens and cook for about 5 minutes.

7. Stir in salt, black pepper, and lemon juice and remove from the heat.

8. Serve hot.

Shrimp Pasta

Ingredients:

- 8 ounces linguine

- ¼ cup mayonnaise

- ¼ cup bean stew glue

- 3 cloves garlic, squashes

- ½ pound shrimp, stripped

- 2 teaspoon salt

- ½ teaspoon cayenne pepper

- 2 teaspoon garlic powder

- 2 tablespoon vegetable oil

- 2 lime, squeezed

- ¼ cup green onion, slashed

- ¼ cup cilantro, minced

- Red bean stew chips, for embellish

Directions:

1. Cook pasta still somewhat firm as per box guidelines. In a little bowl, consolidate mayonnaise, stew glue and garlic.

2. Race to join. Put in a safe spot. In a blending bowl, include shrimp, salt, cayenne and garlic powder.

3. Mix to cover shrimp. Oil in a heavy skillet over medium warmth. Include shrimp and cook for around 2 minutes at that point flip and cook for an extra 2 minutes.

4. Add pasta and sauce to the dish.

5. Mood killer the warmth and combine until the pasta are covered. Include lime, green onions and cilantro, and topped with red bean stew pieces.

Savory Turmeric Pancakes With Lemon Yogurt Sauce

Ingredients:

For the yogurt sauce

- ¼ teaspoon ground turmeric

- 10 fresh mint leaves, minced

- 2 teaspoons lemon zest (from 1 lemon)

- 1 cup plain Greek yogurt

- 1 garlic clove, minced

- 1 to 2 tablespoons lemon juice (from 1 lemon), to taste

For the pancakes

- ½ teaspoon freshly ground black pepper

- 1 head broccoli, cut into florets

- 3 large eggs, lightly beaten

- 2 tablespoons plain unsweetened almond milk

- 1 cup almond flour

- 4 teaspoons coconut oil

- 2 teaspoons ground turmeric

- 1½ teaspoons ground cumin

- 1 teaspoon salt

- 1 teaspoon ground coriander

- ½ teaspoon garlic powder

Directions:

1. Make the yogurt sauce. Combine the yogurt, garlic, lemon juice, turmeric, mint and zest in a bowl. Taste and season with more lemon juice, if required.

2. Reserve or cool till prepared to serve.

3. Make the pancakes. In a small bowl, integrate the turmeric, cumin, salt, coriander, garlic and pepper.

4. Place the broccoli in a food processor, and pulse till the florets are separated into little pieces.

5. Transfer the broccoli to a large bowl and add the eggs, almond milk, and almond flour.

6. Stir in the spice mix and integrate well.

7. Heat 1 teaspoon of the coconut oil in a nonstick pan over medium-low heat.

8. Prepare the pancake until little bubbles begin to appear on the surface and the bottom is golden brown, 2 to 3 minutes.

9. Flip over and cook the pancake for 2 to 3 minutes more.

10. Continue making the staying 3 pancakes, using the staying oil and batter.

Sirt Chilli Con Carne

Ingredients:

- 1 red pepper, cored, seeds removed and cut into bite-sized pieces

- 2 x 400g tins chopped tomatoes

- 1 tbsp tomato purée

- 1 tbsp cocoa powder

- 150g tinned kidney beans

- 300ml beef stock

- 5g coriander, chopped

- 5g parsley, chopped

- 160g buckwheat

- 1 red onion, finely chopped

- 3 garlic cloves, finely chopped

- 2 bird's eye chillies, finely chopped

- 1 tbsp extra virgin olive oil

- 1 tbsp ground cumin

- 1 tbsp ground turmeric

- 400g lean minced beef (5 per cent fat)

- 150ml red wine

Directions:

1. In a casserole, fry the onion, garlic and chilli in the oil over a medium heat for 2-3 minutes, then include the spices and cook for a minute.

2. Add the minced beef and brown over a high heat. Add the red wine and enable it to bubble to reduce it by half.

3. Include the red pepper, tomatoes, tomato purée, cocoa, kidney beans and stock and delegate simmer for 1 hour.

4. You may need to add a little water to accomplish a thick, sticky consistency.

5. Just before serving, stir in the sliced herbs.

6. Cook the buckwheat according to the packet guidelines and serve with the chilli.

Carrot Orange Salad

Ingredients:

- 1 orange

- Salt and pepper

- 1 tsp oregano (chopped)

- 2 cloves of garlic

- 1 tbsp sherry vinegar

- ½ tsp paprika powder

- ½ onion

- 2 tbsp olive oil

- 250 g of carrots

Directions:

1. Wash and dry the orange and grate the zest. Squeeze the juice from the orange and place

in a saucepan with the grated zest and bring
to the boil.

2. Clean, peel and grate the carrots.

3. Then add to the pot and cook until al dente.

4. Chop onion and garlic. Mix in the salt, pepper
   and vinegar.

5. Stir in olive oil and spices. Drain the cooked
   carrots and mix with the sauce.

6. Leave for about an hour.

7. Pour into a salad bowl and serve.

Chinese Cabbage With Apple

Ingredients:

- Small apple

- ½ lemon

- 37 g sour cream

- 125 g chinese cabbage

- 2 tsp olive oil

- 1 toast (whole grain)

- ½ bunch chopped parsley

- 1 teaspoon butter (organic)

- Salt and pepper

Directions:

1. Clean and slice the cabbage.
2. Wash, core and chop the apple into pieces.

3. Add lemon juice.

4. Cut the orange into pieces and collect the juice from the orange.

5. Mix the orange juice with the remaining lemon juice, oil and sour cream. Season with salt and pepper.

6. Cut the whole meal toast into small pieces and fry in a little butter.

7. Arrange the orange pieces, apple and Chinese cabbage in a salad bowl and add the dressing.

8. Refine with the finished toast and parsley.

9. Serve.

Tofu Patties With Mushrooms And Peas

Ingredients:

- 2 tbsp. oil

- 2 cups fresh bean sprouts

- 1 3/4 lbs. tofu, mashed

- 2 tsp. baking powder

- 1 cup flour

- 3 tbsp. nutritional yeast

- 2 tbsp. soy sauce

- 1 cup snow peas

- 1 cup chopped fresh mushrooms

- 8 green onions, chopped

- 1 1/2-inch ginger

- 8 oz. chestnuts, chopped

Directions:

1. Heat a skillet with oil and sauté the onions, mushrooms, snow peas, and chestnuts for 5 to 6 minutes.
2. Add the bean sprouts, mix, and set aside. Remove from heat and set aside. Preheat the oven to 375°F.
3. Blend the tofu and the soy sauce until smooth and creamy.
4. Add flour, nutritional yeast, and baking powder and mix.
5. Add onion, mushrooms, snow peas, and chestnuts.
6. On lined baking tray, form 6 1/2-inch-thick patties.
7. Bake for 30 minutes, flip over and bake for 15 more minutes.

Vanilla Coconut Parfait With Berries

Ingredients:

- 1 cup mixed berries, frozen is perfect

- 1 tbsp. buckwheat granola

- ½ tsp vanilla extract

- 4 oz. coconut yogurt

- 1 tsp agave syrup

Directions:

1. Mix yogurt, vanilla extract, and honey.
2. Alternate yogurt and berries in a jar and top with granola.
3. Frozen berries are perfect if the parfait is made in advance because they release their juices in the yogurt.
4. As far as granola, you can use a tablespoon of the one on this book.

King Prawn Stir-Fry & Soba

Ingredients:

- 1 bird's eye chili, finely chopped

- 1 teaspoon finely chopped fresh ginger

- 20g red onions, sliced

- 40g celery, trimmed and sliced

- 75g green beans, chopped

- 50g kale, roughly chopped

- 100ml chicken stock

- 150g shelled raw king prawns, deveined

- 2 teaspoons tamari

- 2 teaspoons extra virgin olive oil

- 75g soba noddles

- 1 garlic clove, finely chopped

Directions:

1. Warm a skillet over high heat, and then fry the prawns in 1 teaspoon of tamari and 1 teaspoon of olive oil.
2. Transfer the contents of the skillet to a plate, and then wipe the skillet with a kitchen towel to remove the lingering sauce.
3. Boil water and cook the soba for 8 minutes, or according to the package directions.
4. Drain and set aside for later.
5. Using the remaining 1 teaspoon of olive oil, fry the remaining ingredients for 3-4 minutes.
6. Add the stock and bring to a boil, simmering until the vegetables are tender but still have bite.
7. Add the celery, noodles, and prawn into the skillet, stir, bring back to a boil and then serve.

White Clam Sauce

Ingredients:

- 1/2 teaspoon each oregano leaves and salt

- 1 teaspoon white pepper

- 8 ounces drained canned minced clams

- 2 tablespoons chopped fresh parsley

- Serve over cooked linguini or spaghetti.

- 2 teaspoons olive oil

- 1 garlic clove, minced

- 2 cups bottled clam juice

Directions:

1. In 1-quart saucepan heat oil; add garlic and saute just until golden.

2. Add remaining Ingredients: except for clams and parsley and bring to a boil.
3. Reduce heat and let simmer for 5 minutes.
4. Add clams and parsley and cook until thoroughly heated, about 3 minutes longer.

Creole Sauce

Ingredients:

- 1 tablespoon chopped fresh parsley

- 1 cup each diced green bell pepper

- 1/4 teaspoon salt and sliced mushrooms

- Dash pepper

- 1/2 cup chopped celery

- 1 cup canned Italian tomatoes, drained and chopped (reserve liquid)

- 2 teaspoons vegetable oil

- 1 cup canned beef broth

- 1/2 cup diced onion

- 1 bay leaf

- 1 garlic clove, minced

Directions:

1. In 11/2-quart saucepan heat oil; add onion and garlic and saute until onion Is softened.
2. Add green pepper, mushrooms, and celery and saute for 5 minutes.
3. Add tomatoes, reserved liquid, broth, and bay leaf; cover and let simmer for 20 minutes, stirring occasionally.
4. Stir in parsley, salt, and pepper; remove the bay leaf before serving.

Quick Red Bean Stew

Ingredients:

- 1 tsp Mexican seasoning

- 1 tsp hot sauce

- 1 tbsp fresh coriander leaves, for garnishing

- 2 tbsp olive oil

- 1 tbsp cornstarch dissolved in 1 tbsp water

- 1 (14oz/400g) can red beans

- 1 tbsp sweet corn (frozen)

- 1 small red onion, chopped

- 2 cups (500ml) chicken broth

Directions:

1. Heat the olive oil in a small pot and add the onion. Saute for 2 minutes.

2. Add the chicken broth and corn and bring to a boil.
3. Add the red beans, Mexican seasoning, and hot sauce and keep cooking for another 2 minutes.
4. Add the cornstarch and stir to slightly thicken the stew up.
5. Serve in a large bowl and garnish with fresh coriander leaves.

Buckwheat Chocolate Brownies

Ingredients:

- ½ cup (100g) sugar

- 2 eggs

- 1 tbsp cocoa

- 1 tsp vanilla extract

- Greasing spray

- 6 oz (170g) dark chocolate

- ¾ cup (96g) buckwheat flour

- ½ cup unsalted butter

Directions:

1. Preheat the oven to 350F/175C.
2. Mix the buckwheat flour and cocoa in a bowl.

3. Place a heatproof bowl over boiling water (no water inside) and add the dark chocolate and butter to melt.
4. Once melted, remove from the heat.
5. Add the sugar to the melted chocolate and stir well to combine.
6. Add the eggs one at a time while stirring and incorporate them with the buckwheat flour mixture. Add the vanilla extract.
7. Pour the brownie batter in a greased 8X8" baking dish using a spatula and flatten everything up, again using a spatula.
8. Bake in the oven for 25-30 minutes.

Kale And Red Onion Dhal With Buckwheat

Ingredients:

- 1 teaspoon turmeric

- 1 teaspoon garam masala

- 80g red lentils

- 200ml coconut milk

- 100ml water

- 50g kale or spinach

- 80g buckwheat or brown rice

- ½ tablespoon olive oil

- ½ small red onion, sliced

- 1 ½ garlic cloves, crushed

- 1cm ginger, grated

- ½ birds eye chilli, deseeded and finely chopped

Directions:

1. Heat up the olive oil, add the sliced onion and cook on a low heat for 5 minutes until softened with the lid on. Then, add the ginger, garlic, and chilli and continue cooking for extra 1 minute.

2. Add to it, the garam masala, turmeric, and a splash of water. Cook for 1 more minute before adding the coconut milk, red lentils, and 200ml water.

3. Thoroughly mix all together and cook over a gentle heat for 20 minutes with the lid closed. When the dhal starts sticking, add a little more water and stir occasionally.

4. Add the kale, after 20 minutes and thoroughly stir and still cover the lid to cook for additional 5 minutes or 1-2 minutes when you substitute with spinach.

5. Put the buckwheat in a saucepan and pour boiling water like 15 minutes before the curry gets ready. Allow the water to boil and cook for 10-12 minutes.

6. Drain the buckwheat and serve with the dhal.

Char Grilled Beef, A Red Wine Jus, Onion Rings, Garlic Kale

Ingredients:

- 1 garlic clove, finely chopped

- 120–150g x 3.5cm-thick beef fillet steak

- 40ml red wine 150ml beef stock

- 1 teaspoon tomato purée

- 1 teaspoon corn flour

- 1 tablespoon water

- 100g potatoes, peeled and dice

- 1 tablespoon extra virgin olive oil

- 5g parsley, finely chopped

- 50g red onion, sliced into rings

- 50g kale, sliced

Directions:

1. Preheat the oven to 220ºC and put the potatoes in a boiling water and cook for 4–5 minutes, drain.

2. Pour 1 teaspoon oil in a roasting tin and roast the potatoes for 35–45 minutes turning the potatoes on every sides every 10 minutes to ensure they cook evenly.

3. Remove from the oven when fully cooked, sprinkle with chopped parsley and mix thoroughly.

4. Pour 1 teaspoon of the oil on a saucepan and fry the onion for 5-7 minutes to become soft and neatly caramelized. Keep it warm.

5. Place the kale in a saucepan, steam for 2–3 minutes and drain. In ½ teaspoon of oil, fry the garlic for 1 minute to become soft though not coloured.

6. Add the kale and continue to fry for extra 1–2 minutes to become tender. Maintain the warmth.

Spicy Garbanzo And Kale Stew

Ingredients:

- 3 red peppers, chopped

- 2 cups tomato paste

- Salt, ground cayenne pepper and ground cumin to taste

- 2 cups chicken stock

- 4 pounds chicken meat

- 2 cups dry garbanzo beans

- 2 cups chopped onions

- 2 cups kale

- 2 tbsp. olive oil

Directions:

1. Put Ingredients: in the slow cooker. Cover, &
   cook on low for 7 to 9 hours.

Buckwheat Split Pea Soup

Ingredients:

- 3 potatoes, diced

- 1 teaspoon curry powder

- 3 cloves garlic, minced

- ½ cup parsley, chopped

- ½ teaspoon dried oregano

- ½ teaspoon dried thyme

- ½ teaspoon turmeric

- ½ teaspoon black pepper

- 1 tablespoon extra virgin olive oil

- 2 cups dried split peas

- ½ cup buckwheat groats

- 1 ½ teaspoons salt

- 7 cups of water

- 3 carrots, chopped

- 3 stalks celery, chopped

- 1 red onion, diced

Directions:

1. In a large pot, sauté the oil, onion, and garlic for 5 minutes on medium heat, or until garlic is fragrant, and the onions are translucent.
2. Add the peas, buckwheat, salt, and water.
3. Bring just to a boil and then reduce the heat to low. Simmer for 2 hours, stirring occasionally.
4. Add the carrots, celery, red onion, potatoes, dried oregano and thyme, turmeric, and ground black pepper.
5. Simmer for another 45 minutes, or until the peas and vegetables are tender.

6. Add the parsley, stir well and allow to steep for a final 10 minutes.

Hot And Sour Miso Soup

Ingredients:

- 1/4 cup cornstarch

- 1 (8 ounces) container firm tofu, cut into 1/4 inch strips

- 1 (8 ounces) can bamboo shoots, drained

- 1-quart Miso broth

- 1/4 teaspoon chili pepper flakes

- 1 teaspoon ground black pepper

- 1/2 tablespoon chili oil

- 1/2 tablespoon sesame oil

- 1 green onion, sliced

- 6 dried shiitake mushrooms

- 2 cups hot water

- 3 tablespoons soy sauce

- 5 tablespoons rice vinegar

Directions:

1. In a small bowl, place shiitake mushrooms in 1 1/2 cups hot water. Soak for 20 minutes, until rehydrated.
2. Drain, reserving the liquid. Trim stems from the mushrooms and cut into thin strips.
3. In a separate small bowl, blend soy sauce, rice vinegar, and 1 tablespoon cornstarch.
4. Place 1/2 the tofu strips into the mixture.
5. In a medium saucepan, mix the reserved mushroom liquid with the vegetable broth. Bring to a boil and stir in the mushrooms and bamboo shoots.
6. Reduce heat, and simmer 3 to 5 minutes. Season with chili peppers and black pepper.

7. In a small bowl, mix remaining cornstarch and remaining water. Stir into the broth mixture until thickened.

8. Mix soy sauce mixture and remaining tofu strips into the saucepan.

9. Return to boil and stir in the chili oil and sesame oil.

10. Garnish with green onion to serve.

Baked Potatoes With Spicy Chickpea Stew

Ingredients:

- 2 Teaspoons of unsweetened cocoa (or cacao) powder

- 2 Yellow peppers (or any color!), diced in bits of bite size

- Top with salt and pepper (optional)

- 2 Teaspoons of parsley with extra garnish

- Side salad (with option)

- 2 Red onions, shredded

- 2 tbsp. Of olive oil

- 4-6 Baking onions, prickled everywhere

- 4 Cloves, rubbed or ground with garlic

- 1/2 -2 tbsp. Of chilli flakes (depends on how spicy stuff you like)

- 2 cm, dried ginger

- 2 tbsp. Of cumin seeds

- Water-splash

- 2 Spoonful of turmeric

- Tomatoes sliced with 2 x 400 g

- 2 x 400 g tins of chickpeas (or kidney beans, as you like) plus DON'T DRAIN chickpea juice!!

Directions:

1. Oven preheated to 200C, so you can create all the supplies you like.
2. Place the baked potatoes in the oven when it is heated enough, and cook them for 1 hour or when they are cooked as you want them.

3. Put the olive oil and diced red onion into a big broad saucepan until the potatoes are in the oven and cook softly, for 5 minutes with the lid on it, till the onions gets tender but not dark.

4. Remove the cap and add cumin, garlic, ginger and chili.

5. Cook on low heat for another minute, then put the turmeric and a very little water and cook for another minute, and taking some care not letting the saucepan becomes too dry.

6. Next apply cocoa powder (or cacao), chickpea (including chickpea water) and yellow pepper to the tomatoes.

7. Take to boil and cook for 45 minutes at low heat up until the sauce is condensed and dried (but don't burn it!). Stew will be handled nearly at the very same interval as potatoes.

8. Finally, mix in 2 tbsp. parsley, if you like, add some salt and pepper, and place the stew on the top of the roasted potatoes, maybe with basic side salad.

Chickpea, Quinoa And Turmeric Curry Recipe

Ingredients:

- 1 teaspoon ground ginger

- 400g can of coconut milk

- 1 tbsp tomato purée

- 400g can of chopped tomatoes

- Salt and pepper

- 180g quinoa

- 400g can of chickpeas, drained and rinsed

- 150g spinach

- 500g new potatoes, halved

- 3 garlic cloves, crushed

- 3 teaspoons ground turmeric

- 1 teaspoon ground coriander

- 1 teaspoon chilli flakes or powder

Directions:

1. Place the potatoes in a pan of cold water and bring to the boil, then let them cook for about 25 minutes until you can easily stick a knife through them. Drain them well.
2. Place the potatoes in a big pan and include the garlic, turmeric, coriander, chilli, ginger, coconut milk, tomato purée and tomatoes.
3. Give the boil, season with salt and pepper, then include the quinoa with a mug of just-boiled water (300ml).
4. Minimize the heat to a simmer, place the lid on and enable to cook.

5. Over the next 30 minutes, stirring every 5 minutes or so to make sure nothing sticks to the bottom.
6. When there are just 5 minutes left, add the spinach and stir it in up until it wilts.
7. If you like a bit of heat, add a sliced red chilli to the cooking curry at the same time as the other spices.

Turmeric Chicken & Kale Salad With Honey Lime Dressing

Ingredients:

For the chicken

- 1 teaspoon turmeric powder

- 1teaspoon lime zest

- juice of ½ lime

- ½ teaspoon salt + pepper

- 1 teaspoon ghee or 1 tbsp coconut oil

- ½ medium brown onion, diced

- 250-300 g / 9 oz. chicken mince or diced up chicken thighs

- 1 large garlic clove, finely diced

For the salad

- ½ avocado, sliced

- handful of fresh coriander leaves, chopped

- handful of fresh parsley leaves, chopped

- 6 broccoli stalks or 2 cups of broccoli florets

- 2 tablespoons pumpkin seeds (pepitas)

- 3 large kale leaves, stems removed and chopped

For the dressing

- 1 teaspoon raw honey

- ½ teaspoon wholegrain or Dijon mustard

- ½ teaspoon sea salt and pepper

- 3 tablespoons lime juice

- 1 small garlic clove, finely diced or grated

- 3 tablespoons extra-virgin olive oil

Directions:

1. Heat the ghee or coconut oil in a small frying pan over medium-high heat.

2. Add the chicken mince and garlic and stir for 2-3 minutes over medium-high heat, breaking it apart.

3. Add the turmeric, lime zest, lime juice, salt and pepper and cook, stirring often, for a further 3-4 minutes. Set the prepared mince aside.

4. While the chicken is cooking, bring a little pan of water to boil. Add the broccoli and cook for 2 minutes.

5. Include the pumpkin seeds to the fry pan from the chicken and toast over medium heat for 2 minutes, stirring often to prevent burning. Season with a little salt. Reserve.

6. Raw pumpkin seeds are likewise great to use.

7. Place sliced kale in a salad bowl and pour over the dressing.

8. Using your hands, toss and massage the kale with the dressing.

9. This will soften the kale, sort of like what citrus juice does to fish or beef Carpaccio-- it 'cooks' it a little.

10. Toss through the cooked chicken, broccoli, fresh herbs, pumpkin seeds and avocado slices.

Garlic, Spinach, And Chickpea Soup

Ingredients:

- 3 medium potatoes, peeled and chopped

- 1 (15 ounces) can chickpeas, drained

- 1 cup heavy cream

- 2 tablespoons tahini

- 2 tablespoons cornmeal

- 3 cups spinach, rinsed and chopped

- 2 teaspoons fresh parsley, chopped

- Chili pepper flakes to taste

- Salt to taste

- 2 tablespoons olive oil

- 4 cloves garlic, peeled and crushed

- 1 medium yellow onion, coarsely chopped

- 2 teaspoons ground cumin

- 2 teaspoons ground coriander

- 1 1/3 quarts vegetable broth

Directions:

1. Heat olive oil in a large pot over medium heat and stir in garlic and onion.
2. Cook until tender, 2 – 3 minutes. Season with cumin and coriander.
3. Mix vegetable stock and potatoes into the pot and bring to a boil. Reduce heat and simmer about 10 minutes.
4. Stir in the chickpeas and continue to cook until the potatoes are tender about 5 minutes.
5. In a small bowl, blend the heavy cream, tahini, and cornmeal. Mix into the soup.

6. Stir spinach into the soup. Season with parsley, chili pepper flakes, and salt.
7. Continue to cook until spinach is heated through, about another 5 minutes.

Cajun Shrimp Soup

Ingredients:

- 1/4 teaspoon dried basil

- 1/4 teaspoon chili pepper flakes

- 1 bay leaf

- 1/2 teaspoon salt

- 1/2 cup cooked buckwheat groats

- 3/4 pound fresh shrimp, peeled and deveined

- Hot pepper sauce to taste

- 1 tablespoon extra virgin olive oil

- 1/2 cup green bell pepper, chopped

- 1/4 cup green onions, sliced

- 1 clove garlic, minced

- 3 cups tomato juice

- 1 (8 ounces) bottle clam juice

- 1/2 cup water

- 1/4 teaspoon dried lovage

Directions:

1. Warm olive oil in a large pot over medium heat. Sauté bell pepper, onions, and garlic until tender.

2. Stir in tomato juice, clam juice, and water. Season with lovage, basil, chili pepper flakes, bay leaf, and salt.

3. Bring to a boil and stir in buckwheat. Reduce heat and cover. Simmer 15 minutes.

4. Stir in shrimp and cook 5 minutes or until shrimp are opaque.

5. Remove the bay leaf and season with hot sauce to serve.

Tuna, Egg & Caper Salad

Ingredients:

- 2 tomatoes, chopped

- 2 tablespoons fresh parsley, chopped

- 1 red onion, chopped

- 1 stalk of celery

- 1 tablespoon capers

- 2 tablespoons garlic vinaigrette see recipe

- 3½ oz. red chicory or yellow if not available

- 5oz tinned tuna flakes in brine, drained

- 3 ½ oz. cucumber

- 1oz rocket arugula

- 6 pitted black olives

- 2 hard-boiled eggs, peeled and quartered

Directions:

1. Place the tuna, cucumber, olives, tomatoes, onion, chicory, celery, and parsley and rocket arugula into a bowl.
2. Pour in the vinaigrette and toss the salad in the dressing.
3. Serve onto plates and scatter the eggs and capers on top.

Strawberry Buckwheat Pancakes

Ingredients:

- 8fl oz. milk

- 1 teaspoon olive oil

- 1 teaspoon olive oil for frying

- Freshly squeezed juice of 1 orange

- 3½ oz. strawberries, chopped

- 3½ oz. buckwheat flour

- 1 egg

Directions:

1. Pour the milk into a bowl and mix in the egg and a teaspoon of olive oil.
2. Sift in the flour to the liquid mixture until smooth and creamy.

3. Allow it to rest for 15 minutes. Heat a little oil in a pan and pour in a quarter of the mixture or to the size you prefer.
4. Sprinkle in a quarter of the strawberries into the batter.
5. Cook for around 2 minutes on each side.
6. Serve hot with a drizzle of orange juice.
7. You could try experimenting with other berries such as blueberries and blackberries.

Buckwheat Noodles With Chicken Kale

Ingredients:

For the noodles

- 1 teaspoon coconut oil or ghee

- 1 brown onion, finely diced

- 1 medium free-range chicken breast, sliced or diced

- 1 long red chilli, thinly sliced (seeds in or out depending on how hot you like it)

- 2 large garlic cloves, finely diced

- 2-3 tablespoons Tamari sauce (gluten-free soy sauce)

- 2-3 handfuls of kale leaves (removed from the stem and roughly cut)

- 150 g / 5 oz buckwheat noodles (100% buckwheat, no wheat)

- 3-4 shiitake mushrooms, sliced

For the miso dressing

- 1 tablespoon extra-virgin olive oil

- 1 tablespoon lemon or lime juice

- 1 teaspoon sesame oil (optional)

- 1½ tablespoon fresh organic miso

- 1 tablespoon Tamari sauce

Directions:

1. Add the kale and cook for 1 minute, until a little wilted.
2. Get rid of and set aside but book the water and bring it back to the boil.

3. Include the soba noodles and cook according to the plan guidelines (typically about 5 minutes).

4. In the meantime, pan fry the shiitake mushrooms in a little ghee or coconut oil (about a teaspoon) for 2-3 minutes, up until lightly browned on each side. Sprinkle with sea salt and reserved.

5. Cook 5 minutes over medium heat, stirring a couple of times, then include the garlic, tamari sauce and a little splash of water.

6. Cook for a more 2-3 minutes, stirring frequently up until chicken is prepared through.

7. Finally, include the kale and soba noodles and toss through the chicken to warm up.

8. Mix the miso dressing and drizzle over the noodles right at the end of cooking, by doing this you will keep all those beneficial probiotics in the miso alive and active.

Onion Salad With Cherry Tomatoes

Ingredients:

- 6 cherry tomatoes

- 1 red onion

- 1 clove of garlic

- Salt and pepper

- 2 tbsp olive oil

- Chopped parsley (1 bunch)

Directions:

1. Wash and halve the cherry tomatoes.
2. Peel the onion and cut into rings.
3. Wash and chop the parsley and place in a bowl with the tomatoes and onion. Chop the garlic cloves and add.

4. Finally stir in the oil. Season with salt and pepper.

Quick Onion Salad

Ingredients:

- 1 tsp chili flakes

- Bit of apple cider vinegar

- ½ bunch of parsley

- 2 onions

- 2 tbsp olive oil

- Salt

- Pepper

Directions:

1. Peel and slice the onions and place in a salad bowl.

2. Add the remaining Ingredients: and mix everything together.
3. Leave for about an hour.
4. A very light and healthy appetizer. Good Appetite.

Baked Eggplant With Turmeric And Garlic

Ingredients:

- 1/4 tsp. Turmeric

- 1/4 cup water

- 2 tbsp. White poppy seeds made into a paste

- 1/2 tsp. Salt

- 1/2 tsp. Sugar

- Eggplant

- 2 tbsp. Extra-virgin olive oil

- 2 chilies

- 1 1/2 tbsp. Garlic, diced

- 1 tsp. Green chili

Directions:

1. Crush the poppy seeds with a drop of olive oil to form a paste.

2. Preheat oven to 450°F. Cut eggplant lengthwise and place it on a baking sheet with the cut side down.

3. Bake for 30 to 34 minutes or until the eggplant wrinkles and feels soft to the touch when pressed. Cut.

4. Set aside. Heat a skillet with oil over medium heat. Fry red chilies until they are soft.

5. Add garlic and green chili. Stir until garlic turns light brown.

6. Add water and turmeric and bring to a boil.

7. Lower the heat and stir in the eggplant cuts.

8. Add poppy seed paste, salt, and sugar and mix well.

9. Simmer covered for 20 minutes, occasionally stirring.

10. Trim with green onions and serve.

Banana Berry Kale Smoothie

Ingredients:

- 1 cup kale (chopped)

- 1 cup ice

- 1 banana

- 1 cup strawberries (fresh or frozen)

Directions:

1. Add all Ingredients: to a high-power blender and pulse until smooth.
2. Pour the smoothie into two glasses and serve immediately.
3. It can be stored in the refrigerator in an airtight container for up to 3 days.

Roasted Sardines With Parsley

Ingredients:

- 1 teaspoon black pepper

- 1 garlic clove, crushed

- 2 tablespoons white wine

- 1 tablespoon extra-virgin olive oil

- 400 g fresh sardines already cleaned

- 2 lemons zest

- Salt

- 50 g chopped parsley

Directions:

1. Prepare the sauce by blending the parsley, pepper, garlic clove and thinly grated lemon zest. Also add the white wine, lemon juice and oil.

2. Cook the sardines in a non-stick pan (or grill) for one minute per side.
3. When serving, pour a little sauce on the plate, lay the sardines on top and season with other sauce.
4. Complete with a pinch of salt and lemon zest cut into strips.

Chicken Fry With Peanut Sauce

Ingredients:

- 1 garlic clove, minced

- 1 teaspoon powdered ginger

- 1-2 teaspoons hot sauce, if desired

- 2 red bell peppers, chopped

- 2 tablespoons toasted sesame seeds

- 4 green onions, thinly sliced

- Meat from 4 chicken thighs, cut into bite-size pieces

- 2 tablespoons + ¼ cup peanut oil

- ½ cup peanut butter

- 3 tablespoons toasted sesame oil

- 2 tablespoons soy sauce

- 1 tablespoon lime juice

Directions:

1. Heat 2 tablespoons of peanut oil in a large frying pan.
2. Add the chicken and cook for about 10 minutes, until no pink remains.
3. Meanwhile, mix together the peanut butter, ¼ cup peanut oil, sesame oil, soy sauce, lime juice, garlic, ginger, and hot sauce.
4. Add more water if needed to achieve a smooth consistency.
5. When the chicken is done, add the red pepper and cook for 1 more minute.
6. Divide the chicken and peppers between four plates and top with peanut sauce, toasted sesame seeds, and green onions.

Tartar Sauce

Ingredients:

- 1 teaspoon each Worcestershire sauce and lemon juice

- 1 tablespoon pickle relish

- 1 teaspoon chopped drained capers

- 2 teaspoon chopped fresh parsley

- Delicious with fish.

- 1/4 cup reduced-calorie mayonnaise

- 1 teaspoon Dijon-style mustard

Directions:

1. In small bowl mix mayonnaise with mustard, Worcestershire sauce, and lemon juice; stir in pickle relish, capers, and parsley. Serve

immediately or cover and refrigerate until ready to serve

Crust less Asparagus Quiche

Ingredients:

- 2 eggs, beaten

- 2 ounces shredded Swiss cheese, divided

- 1/4 teaspoon pepper

- Dash each salt and ground red pepper

- 2 teaspoons margarine, divided

- 1/4 cup chopped scallions (green onions)

- 1 cup cooked chopped asparagus (1/2-inch pieces)

- 1/2 cup evaporated skimmed milk

Directions:

1. Preheat oven to 375°F.

2. In small skillet heat 1 teaspoon margarine
    until bubbly and hot; add scallions and saute
    until softened.

3. In a medium bowl, combine sautéed scallions
    with asparagus, milk, eggs, 1-ounce cheese,
    and the seasonings.

4. Grease 7-inch pie plate with remaining
    teaspoon margarine and pour in egg mixture;
    sprinkle with remaining 1-ounce cheese and
    bake for 35 minutes (until a knife, inserted In
    the center, comes out clean).

Bacon-Wrapped Filled Dates

Ingredients:

- 12 thin slices of streaky bacon, cut in half

- 2 tbsp roasted almonds, roughly chopped

- 20 dates, pitted and torn halfway

- 2 tbsp ricotta or cream cheese

Directions:

1. Take a small piping bag and fill it with the ricotta cheese. Fill the dates with the ricotta cheese.
2. Wrap one (half) bacon slice over each date and secure with a toothpick.
3. Transfer to a baking tray lined with parchment paper and bake at 420F/215C for 20 minutes.
4. Serve with the toasted almonds.

Matcha Coconut Pudding

Ingredients:

- ¼ cup (50g) white sugar

- 3 tbsp green bean paste missed

- Whipping cream (optional)

- 1 ½ tbsp Matcha powder, sifted

- 2 gelatin sheets or 10g gelatin powder

- 1 ¼ cup (300 ml) warm milk

- 2 tbsp water

Directions:

1. Cut the gelatin sheets (if applicable) into thin strips and add the 2 tbsp water in a bowl.
2. Heat the gelatin-water using a double boiler (bowl over a pot of boiling water) to dissolve.

3. Once dissolved, take off the heat and keep it aside.
4. Bring the milk to a boil and remove from the heat.
5. Add the sugar and whisk well to dissolve.
6. Add a few tablespoons of the milk mixture to the sifted matcha powder and stir to dissolve.
7. Add the match mixture back to the remaining milk and stir well.
8. Add the green paste, stir and add the gelatin. Stir well.
9. Distribute the mixture into 4 glass containers, let chill, and keep in the fridge for at least 3 hours.
10. Add a bit of whipping cream on top (optionally) to garnish.

Buckwheat Pasta Salad

Ingredients:

- 8 cherry tomatoes, halved

- 1/2 avocado, diced

- 10 olives

- 1 tablespoon extra virgin olive oil

- 20g pine nuts

- 50g buckwheat pasta

- Large handful of rocket

- Small handful of basil leaves

Directions:

1. Cook the pasta according to the packet
   Directions: and set aside

2. Apart from the pine nut, combine all the Ingredients: including the cooked pasta and arrange on a plate or in a bowl.

3. Scatter the pine nuts all over the top. Enjoy.

Greek Salad Skewers

Ingredients:

- 1 yellow pepper

- ½ red onion, chopped

- 100g cucumber, sliced

- 100g feta, chopped into 8

- 2 wooden skewers

- 8 large black olives

- 8 cherry tomatoes

For the dressing

- 1 tablespoon of extra virgin olive oil

- ½ lemon

- 1 teaspoon of balsamic vinegar

- ½ clove garlic, peeled and crushed

- Few basil leaves, finely chopped

- Few leaves oregano, finely chopped

- Salt

- Freshly ground black pepper

Directions:

1. Soaked the wooden skewers in water for 30 minutes before use.

2. Thread each skewer with the salad Ingredients: in the order: olive, tomato, yellow pepper, red onion, cucumber, feta, tomato, olive, yellow pepper, red onion, cucumber, feta.

3. Put the entire dressing Ingredients: in a bowl and mix together vigorously. Pour over the skewers.

Garbanzo Kale Curry

Ingredients:

- 1 cup sliced tomato

- 2 cups kale leaves

- 1/2 cup coconut milk

- 4 cups dry garbanzo beans

- Curry Paste, but go low on the heat

Directions:

1. Put Ingredients: in the slow cooker.
2. Cover, & cook on low for 7 to 9 hours.

Exotic Muesli With Tropical Fruits

Ingredients:

- 100 g coconut muesli (finished product)

- 200 ml of coconut water (tetra-pack)

- 1 small papaya

- 1 kiwi

- 1 persimmon not too ripe

Directions:

1. Halve the papaya, remove the seeds with a spoon, and peel the papaya. Finely dice the pulp.
2. Peel the kiwi with the peeler and dice the pulp.
3. Wash the persimmon, cut out the stem and dice the pulp.

4. Put the cereal and fruit in bowls and pour the coconut water over them.

Spicy Mango Salad With Sheep's Cheese

Ingredients:

- 300 g small, ripe mango (1 small, ripe mango)

- 4th culms of chives

- 1 stem

- Basil

- ½ organic lemon

- Pepper from the mill

- 10 g sheep cheese (9% absolute fat)

Directions:

1. Wash the mango, rub dry and peel with a peeler.

2. Cut the flesh from the stone in thick slices, dice, and place in a bowl.

3. Wash herbs and shake dry. Cut the chives into rolls.
4. Pluck the basil leaves, put some aside, and cut the rest into fine strips.
5. Squeeze the lemon, add the juice with chives and basil strips to the mango cubes.
6. Season with pepper and let steep for 10 minutes.
7. Arrange the mango salad. Dab the sheep cheese dry with kitchen paper and crumble it over the salad with your fingers. Garnish with basil leaves.